RFK JR.
WILL FAIL!
WITHOUT
THIS CRITICAL PIECE

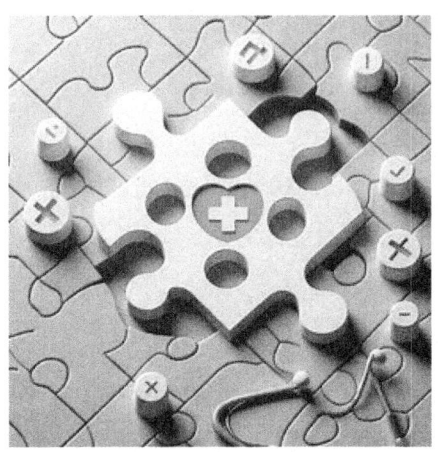

OF THE PUZZLE!

Jeff T Bowles

Table of Contents:

Introduction: 5
Historical Errors and Misconceptions 6
The IOM's Decimal Point Error 6
Debunking Vitamin D3 Toxicity Myths 7
The Importance of Cofactors: 9
The Crucial Role of Magnesium 9
Vitamin K2 and Other Cofactors 10
Vitamin D3 and Health: 12
The Latitude Effect on Autoimmune Diseases & Cancer . 12
Bone Health 14
Type 2 Diabetes 15
The Human Antifreeze System 19
Implications for Modern Health 21
Did Humans Really Hibernate? 21
Recent Evidence of Human Hibernation 21
The Two Systems of Vitamin D3 Metabolism 22
Endocrine System 22
Autocrine/Paracrine System 23
The Misunderstanding and Its Consequences 23
Skyrocketing Incidence of Diseases Since the 1980s 27
Remarkable Results of High-Dose 34
Vitamin D3 Supplementation 34
Autoimmune Diseases: The Coimbra Protocol 34
Cancer Prevention and Treatment 36

Cardiovascular Health 37
Neurological Conditions 37
Metabolic Health 37
Immune Function and Infection Resistance 39
Mental Health 40
Safety and Monitoring 41
Remarkable Results of High-Dose Vitamin D3 Supplementation 42
Anecdotal Cancer Cases 42
Prostate Cancer Research by Dr. Bruce Hollis 43
Vitamin D3 and Mitochondrial Function 45
The COVID-19 Pandemic and Vitamin D3 48
Suppression of Vitamin D3 Information 50
False Information 52
The VITAL Study: A Flawed Approach to Vitamin D3 Research 57
Misinterpretation of Results: Ignoring Positive Findings ..59
Overlooking Cofactors: The Magnesium Connection 61
The Latitude Effect: A Missed Opportunity 62
Beyond Bone Health: Vitamin D's Multifaceted Role 63
The Need for Personalized Approaches 63
Reinterpreting VITAL: A Call for Nuanced Analysis 65
Moving Forward: Recommendations for Future Research 67
Cancer Prevention and Mortality 71
Practical Implications: What This Means for Public Health
....71
A Call for Critical Thinking 72

Summary of Dr. Clifford Rosen's Editorial About the
VITAL Study 74
Biologics: A Double-Edged Sword 76
The Ultimate Biologic: Vitamin D3 77
The Hostility of Big Medicine 78
The Suppression of Vitamin D: A Historical Perspective . 79
Ongoing Conspiracy? 81
Conclusion: The Vitamin D3 Revolution - Unveiling the
Truth and Transforming Health 87
Appendix A- Fixing our Soils 93
The Hidden Epidemic: Soil Mineral Deficiencies 93
A Soil Restoration Plan for RFK Jr.? 96
Appendix B- Either Outlaw the Feeding of Corn 100
to Our Livestock or Require Fortification 100
A proposed plan to address the vitamin K2 issue: 106
Proposed Plan for Nationwide Implementation 108

Introduction:

Shocking Ignorance Surrounding Vitamin D3

The medical and scientific communities have long underestimated or suppressed the importance of vitamin D3, leading to widespread deficiency and numerous health issues. This ignorance stems from a series of possibly deliberate promotions of misconceptions, errors, and outdated information that continue to influence public health policies and medical practices.

Vitamin D3 is NOT a Vitamin!

The definition of vitamin is a substance that your body cannot make itself and you need to get it through your diet. When vitamin D was discovered, it was thought to be an essential vitamin that was found in cod liver oil because when cod liver oil was added to dogs' food (who were raised wholly indoors) they did not get rickets -a disease that deforms the bones of the legs in a bowing pattern.

Because vitamin C was the last vitamin to be discovered, they named this new substance found in cod liver oil vitamin D.

A subsequent experiment showed that dogs raised outdoors and fed the same diet as the prior experimental dogs, except that they did not eat cod liver oil, did **not** get rickets. Somehow the sun exposure protected them from the bone disease.

It turns out that the dogs made vitamin D3 in their skin and fur just by sitting in the sun. Because they could make it themselves, by definition, vitamin D3 is not a vitamin.

So, then what is it?
Vitamin D3 is actually a steroid hormone (made from chole**sterol**) that, by some estimates, controls or influences 2,700+ of the roughly 20,000 genes in the human genome.

Historical Errors and Misconceptions

The IOM's Decimal Point Error
One of the most egregious mistakes concerning vitamin D3 since 400 IUs per day was set as the daily recommended dose in 1940, came from the Institute of Medicine (IOM) in 2011. They made a critical decimal point error in calculating the daily dosage, recommending a mere 600 to 800 IU of vitamin D3 per day.
(Although this new recommendation was an increase from 400 IUs per day which had been

the recommended daily dose since the 1940, 600 to 800 IUs a day was still outrageously low).

This error(?) led to a severe underestimation of the body's vitamin D3 needs.
In reality, the correct daily dosage should be 8,000 to 10,000 IU per day – more than ten times the amount initially recommended. This was calculated and confirmed by two separate research teams who audited and reevaluated IOM's erroneous calculations. To put this into perspective, 10,000 IU of vitamin D3 is equivalent to the amount produced by the skin (light-pigmented skin) during just 15 minutes of sunbathing. This natural production capacity highlights how far off the mark current recommendations are from the body's actual needs.

Debunking Vitamin D3 Toxicity Myths

Contrary to popular belief, there is no such thing as vitamin D3 toxicity in the traditional sense. What is often misdiagnosed as "toxicity" is actually an induced deficiency in vitamin D3's cofactors, primarily magnesium and vitamin K2. (And to a lesser extent boron, zinc, and vitamin A).
- Magnesium Deficiency: High-dose vitamin D3 supplementation can quickly deplete

magnesium stores, leading to symptoms in already-magnesium-deficient people that may be mistaken for vitamin D3 toxicity such as heart racing, dizziness, falls, blood pressure changes, constipation, muscle cramps, insomnia, panic attacks, confusion and many more, even including convulsions, hallucinations and death.

- Vitamin K2 Deficiency: While extremely rare, longer-term high-dose vitamin D3 (in the range of hundreds of thousands of IUs per day) can lead to hypercalcemia typically after about six months of taking 100,000's of IUs per day if not balanced with adequate vitamin K2. Vitamin K2 is essential for removing calcium from the blood and putting it back into the bones where it belongs. If vitamin D3 depletes most of one's K2 stores, then soft tissues can become calcified and hypercalcemia (excess calcium in the blood) might also result. Feeding extremely high doses of D3 without K2 to rats is what allows vitamin D3 to be used as rat poison. If enough K2 was added to the D3-rat poison, the rats would probably not be affected.

The Importance of Cofactors:

The Crucial Role of Magnesium

A critical aspect of vitamin D3 metabolism that is often overlooked is the role of magnesium. A review published in The Journal of the American Osteopathic Association found that vitamin D can't be metabolized without sufficient magnesium levels, meaning vitamin D remains stored and inactive for as many as 80 percent of the magnesium deficient Americans.
People are taking vitamin D supplements but don't realize how it gets metabolized. Without magnesium, vitamin D is not nearly as effective.

It is of the utmost importance to maintain adequate magnesium levels alongside vitamin D3 supplementation. Foods high in magnesium include legumes, nuts, seeds, green leafy vegetables, whole grains, and some dairy products. **However,** because modern farming practices have depleted most soils of magnesium as well as boron and zinc, supplementation is almost a requirement to achieve proper magnesium levels in today's world. Some estimate that 80%+ of the population is magnesium deficient which remains undetected because doctors do not have any useful test for it. Real testing would require muscle and tissue biopsies to measure the magnesium in the body. Only 1% of the body's magnesium is found in the blood and its level is tightly controlled. This makes the magnesium blood test basically worthless as a diagnostic tool. Magnesium deficiencies exist in the various tissues and bones and can take up to a year to reverse with an intensive magnesium supplementation program.

Vitamin K2 and Other Cofactors

Vitamin K2's primary function is to activate specific proteins that regulate calcium in the body.

When K2 is deficient:
1. Osteocalcin remains inactive, preventing proper calcium deposition in bones and teeth
2. Matrix-GLA protein is not activated, failing to prevent calcium from accumulating in soft tissues
3. This leads to a paradoxical situation where bones become weaker while arteries and other soft tissues become calcified
4. The body's ability to regulate calcium metabolism is severely impaired, affecting multiple organ systems

Taking higher doses of vitamin D3 can eventually deplete one's vitamin K2 stores leading to K2 deficiency symptoms like hypercalcemia which many doctors call vitamin D toxicity. By ensuring adequate K2 intake, many of these health issues can potentially be prevented or mitigated. It's important to note that K2 works synergistically with other nutrients, particularly vitamins D3 and A, so a balanced approach to nutrition is key for optimal health. Many people taking both vitamin D3 and k2 at higher doses have reported that calcification in their veins and arteries just disappeared often within a year- surprising their doctors. Also, in one study in Japan, 45 mg/day of K2 was given to women with osteoporosis and this was found to be an effective treatment for it. See: Vitamin K2 Therapy for Postmenopausal Osteoporosis Nutrients 2014 May 16;6(5):1971–1980. Jun Iwamoto 1

Taking very high doses of vitamin D3, K2, and magnesium for an extended period without adequate intake of other essential cofactors like boron and zinc could potentially lead to several other health issues:
Prolonged high-dose vitamin D3 supplementation without sufficient zinc intake may result in:

- Impaired immune function, leading to increased susceptibility to infections
- Delayed wound healing and skin problems
- Altered taste and smell perception
- Potential impact on vitamin D metabolism, as zinc acts as a cofactor for vitamin D-dependent gene transcription

Boron Deficiency

While less studied than zinc, boron deficiency in the context of high vitamin D3 intake might lead to:

- Reduced effectiveness of vitamin D, as boron is believed to enhance vitamin D metabolism
- Potential negative impacts on bone health, as boron plays a role in calcium metabolism
- Arthritis (To be discussed in detail later)

Vitamin D3 and Health:

The Latitude Effect on Autoimmune Diseases & Cancer

One of the most intriguing aspects of vitamin D3 research is the "latitude effect" observed in autoimmune disease and cancer rates (and other diseases). Epidemiological studies have consistently shown that people living at southern latitudes, where sunlight exposure is higher, have much lower rates of autoimmune diseases and cancer compared to those living at northern latitudes. This observation led researchers to believe that variation in vitamin D levels, which are influenced by sunlight exposure, account for these disease associations.

Incidence of Multiple Sclerosis in 55 Countries-
X axis = Latitude
Y axis = Incidence of MS per 100,000 population

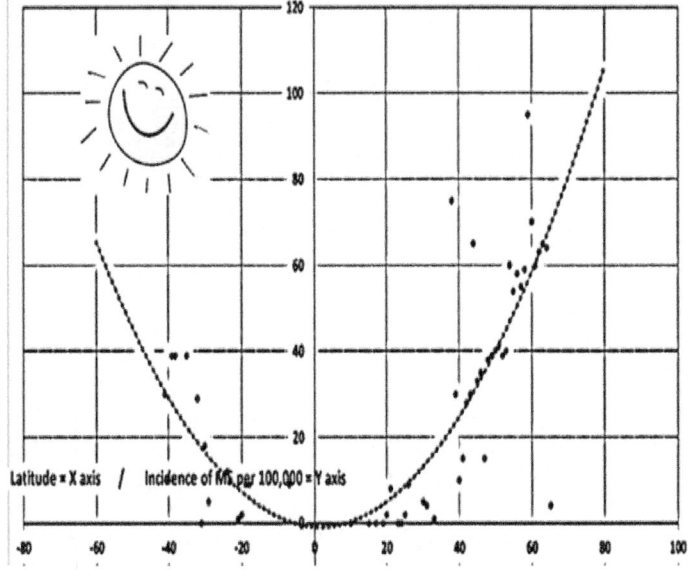

You will see this happy face distribution for virtually every autoimmune disease and every form of cancer as well as asthma and many other diseases. All you have to do is go to your favorite search engine (I prefer the less censored

BING search engine) and type in the disease of interest, and the terms "latitude" and "incidence" and then look at the images that pop up. You will get almost the exact same "smiley face" graph you see above over and over.

Bone Health

While the primary focus of vitamin D3 has traditionally been on bone health, recent large-scale studies have shown mixed results:
1. The VITAL study did not find a protective effect from vitamin D supplements on bone fractures in healthy adults. (You will later see that the VITAL study is a designed-to-fail junk-science study intended to persuade the public to not take vitamin D3 supplements).

2. However, other studies have shown that vitamin D and calcium supplementation can modestly decrease the risk of major fractures in older adults with poor vitamin D status or calcium intake. (I do NOT recommend taking extra calcium with higher dose vitamin D3-you get plenty from your diet).

Type 2 Diabetes

The D2d study, which evaluated the effects of daily vitamin D supplementation (4,000 IU per day) on the conversion of prediabetes to type 2 diabetes mellitus (T2DM), found some promising results:
1. While the overall effect was not statistically significant, a post hoc analysis showed a significant effect in individuals with
   - a baseline body mass index below 30 mg/m^2,
     (larger people need larger doses of D3)
   - severe vitamin D deficiency at baseline,
   - perfect adherence to treatment during the study, or
   - serum 25(OH)D above 40 ng/ml throughout the study
2. A meta-analysis of multiple trials concluded that vitamin D supplementation decreased the risk of progression to T2DM by about 10%, especially when using doses above 1,000 IU per day and in participants without obesity.

I have heard many anecdotal reports from people taking much higher doses of vitamin D3 (40,000 IUs + per day) that they were able to significantly reduce or eliminate their diabetes medications typically after about 6 months of treatment. You can read about these various cases by using the Search D3 cures- search engine here:

https://jefftbowles.com/vitamin-d3-cure-search-engine-can-d3-cure-your-disease-1000-case-studies/

Why Would Evolution Create Such a System? Why Not Just Stimulate Vitamin D3 Receptors All the Time and Get Rid of Cancer and So Many Other Diseases?

The Human Hibernation Syndrome
The Human Hibernation Syndrome is an idea I came up with after wondering why evolution would want us to get sick and diseased in the winter? After some thought it occurred to me that it might be an evolutionary adaptation that allowed our ancestors to survive periods of food scarcity and harsh winter conditions. The key points of this hypothetical syndrome include:

1. Vitamin D3 as a seasonal signal: Decreasing levels of vitamin D3, typically associated with reduced sunlight exposure in winter, triggers the body to prepare for potential famine and cold temperatures.

2. Metabolic changes: The body responds to low vitamin D3 levels by:
    - Increasing appetite and fat storage (similar to bears where a 70% decline in seasonal D3 levels lead to voracious overeating and an increase from summer weight by 70% prior to hibernating.)
    - Slowing down metabolism
    - Inducing depression to conserve energy
    - Potentially increasing susceptibility to common colds to keep one house (cave) bound to further conserve energy
    - Temporarily inducing a large variety of autoimmune diseases meant to keep one house (cave) bound to conserve energy

3. Incomplete Repair Syndrome: The body conserves resources by only partially repairing injuries and performing minimal

maintenance, leading to accumulation of health issues over time.

The Human Antifreeze System

From the Human Hibernation Syndrome emerged a sub theory which I call the "Human Antifreeze System" that is activated in response to low vitamin D3 levels. This system is designed to help the body survive freezing temperatures that would normally crystallize blood and damage tissues. The key components of this system include:

1. Increased blood sugar: The development of type II diabetes-like conditions raises blood sugar levels, which lowers the freezing point of blood, similar to how ethylene glycol (a sugar) acts as antifreeze in cars.
2. Elevated blood pressure: High blood pressure causes more gases to dissolve in the blood, further lowering its freezing point.
3. Glaucoma: The increased pressure in the eye fluids is another manifestation of the antifreeze system, helping to prevent freezing of the non-circulating intra ocular fluid.
4. Salt craving: Rather than salt causing high blood pressure for which there is limited, unpersuasive evidence, I suggest that

people with high blood pressure crave salt as an additional antifreeze mechanism for the blood. We put salt on roads and walks in the winter to lower the freezing temperature of water and melt the ice. Increased salt in the blood and tissues may also lower freezing points.

5. Other tissues damaged by diabetes: kidneys, eyes, ears, feet, fingers. All tissues more susceptible to freezing damage either by being far from the core of the body, more likely to be exposed, or filled with non-circulating fluids. I expect these tissues will all be found to have higher concentrations of sugar than other body parts in diabetics.

Evolutionary Rationale

I believe that these systems evolved to enhance survival during periods of extreme cold and resource scarcity. The ability to lower the freezing point of bodily fluids and slow metabolism would have provided a significant survival advantage for early humans facing long, harsh winters with limited food availability.

Implications for Modern Health

If this is true, many modern health issues, including autoimmune diseases, cancer, obesity, depression, type II diabetes, high blood pressure, glaucoma, and even autism, bipolar disease and many others may be unintended consequences of our bodies' ancient survival mechanisms being activated inappropriately due to chronic vitamin D3 deficiency.

Did Humans Really Hibernate?
Recent Evidence of Human Hibernation

Interestingly, recent research provides some support for the idea of human hibernation. A study published in the journal Anthropology in 2020 examined fossilized bones from the Sima de loss Hueso's cave in northern Spain, dating back approximately 400,000 years. The

researchers found evidence suggesting that these early humans may have entered a hibernation-like state to survive harsh winters:
1. Bone lesions: The fossils showed signs of lesions and bone damage indicative of conditions like hyperparathyroidism, which are often associated with hibernation in other mammals. (High dose vitamin D3 suppresses parathyroid hormone production).
2. Seasonal growth patterns: The bones displayed evidence of annual growth disruptions, similar to those seen in hibernating species.
3. Environmental context: The individuals lived during a period of extreme glaciation, where hibernation could have been a crucial survival strategy.

The Two Systems of Vitamin D3 Metabolism

Endocrine System
The endocrine system, which has been the primary focus of vitamin D research for decades, is responsible for maintaining bone health and calcium homeostasis. In this system:
- Vitamin D3 is converted to 25-hydroxyvitamin D [25(OH)D] in the liver.
- 25(OH)D has a half-life of approximately three weeks in circulation.

- 25(OH)D is further converted to 1,25-dihydroxyvitamin D [1,25(OH)2D] in the kidneys for endocrine function.

Autocrine/Paracrine System

The autocrine/paracrine system, extensively researched by the great Dr. Bruce Hollis, has been less appreciated until recently, involves:
- Direct delivery of vitamin D3 to all tissues of the body.
- Local conversion of vitamin D3 to its active form within cells of various tissues.
- **A much shorter half-life of approximately 24 hours** for vitamin D3 in this system.

The Misunderstanding and Its Consequences

Many researchers have focused solely on the endocrine system, neglecting the importance of the autocrine/paracrine system. This oversight has led to several problematic assumptions and practices:
1. Infrequent Dosing: Researchers often design studies with weekly, monthly, or even yearly vitamin D3 supplementation, assuming that the long half-life of 25(OH)D in the endocrine system is sufficient for all vitamin D functions.

2. Neglect of Daily Requirements: The autocrine system's need for daily vitamin D3 replenishment is overlooked, potentially compromising immune function and other non-skeletal benefits of vitamin D3.
3. Misinterpretation of Results: Studies using infrequent dosing fail to capture the full benefits of vitamin D3, particularly in areas related to immune function and disease prevention
4. With respect to using vitamin D3 to treat COVID 19 one Brazilian study found that a single dose of 200,000 IUs of regular D3 (cholecalciferol) upon admission to the ICU failed to improve the outcome of Covid 19 patients. However, a Spanish study that gave 50 patients every- other-day dosing of activated vitamin D3 (calcifediol a more active form of D3) saw a reduction in ICU admissions vs controls by 96% and a 100% decline in deaths vs. controls.

Impact on Research and Clinical Trials
This misunderstanding has led to numerous studies that may be considered "worthless" or misleading for several reasons:
1. Inadequate Dosing Frequency: Studies using weekly, monthly, or yearly doses fail to maintain consistent levels of vitamin D3 for the autocrine system, potentially missing its benefits for immune function and other non-skeletal health outcomes.
2. Focus on Total 25(OH)D Levels: Many studies rely solely on measuring total serum 25(OH)D levels, which may not accurately reflect the availability of vitamin D3 for autocrine functions.
3. Neglect of Free Vitamin D: The importance of free (unbound) vitamin D3 and 25(OH)D, which are more readily available for cellular uptake and autocrine functions, is often overlooked.
4. Failure to Consider Vitamin D Binding Protein (DBP): The role of DBP in regulating the availability of free vitamin D metabolites is frequently not accounted for in study designs.
5. Disregard for Individual Variations: Genetic differences in vitamin D metabolism and binding protein levels are often not considered, leading to one-size-

fits-all approaches that may not be effective for all individuals.

Implications for Future Research and Clinical Practice

To address these issues and conduct more meaningful vitamin D3 research:
1. Daily Dosing: Studies should prioritize daily vitamin D3 supplementation to maintain consistent levels for both endocrine and autocrine function.
2. Measurement of Free Vitamin D: Assessing free vitamin D3 and 25(OH)D levels, in addition to total 25(OH)D, may provide a more accurate picture of vitamin D status.
3. Consideration of Genetic Factors: Accounting for individual variations in vitamin D metabolism and binding protein levels could lead to more personalized and effective supplementation strategies.
4. Focus on Non-Skeletal Outcomes: More attention should be given to studying the effects of vitamin D3 on immune function, autoimmune diseases, and other non-skeletal health outcomes.
5. Longer-Term Studies: Given the potential for cumulative effects of daily vitamin D3

supplementation, longer-term studies may be necessary to fully capture its benefits.

By addressing these issues and adopting a more nuanced understanding of vitamin D3 metabolism, future research can provide more accurate and useful insights into the role of vitamin D3 in human health, potentially leading to more effective supplementation strategies and improved health outcomes.

Skyrocketing Incidence of Diseases Since the 1980s

What follows is a summary of the reported increase in various diseases and conditions since the 1980s, which I attribute to increased sunscreen use and sun avoidance practices purportedly to reduce the incidence of basal call and squamous cell skin cancer-the easily treatable kind. At the same time melanoma rates have skyrocketed! Melanoma is the deadly kind of skin cancer that appears usually on skin not exposed to the sun like palms of hand or soles of feet.

Sunscreen and sun avoidance just so happened to dramatically reduce the population's vitamin D3 levels, an innocent oversight? You be the judge:

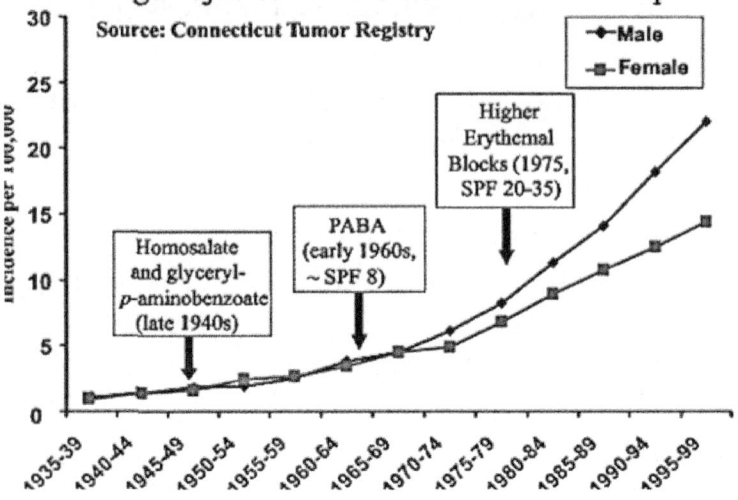

Dates of introduction of suntan lotions and sunscreens and age-adjusted melanoma incidence rates per 100,000

Autoimmune Diseases
1. Multiple Sclerosis (MS):
    - Incidence has reportedly doubled since the 1980s in many regions.
    - Particularly notable increases in northern latitudes with less sunlight exposure.
2. Type 1 Diabetes:
    - Significant increase, especially in children under 5 years old.
    - Some studies report a 3-5% annual increase in incidence.

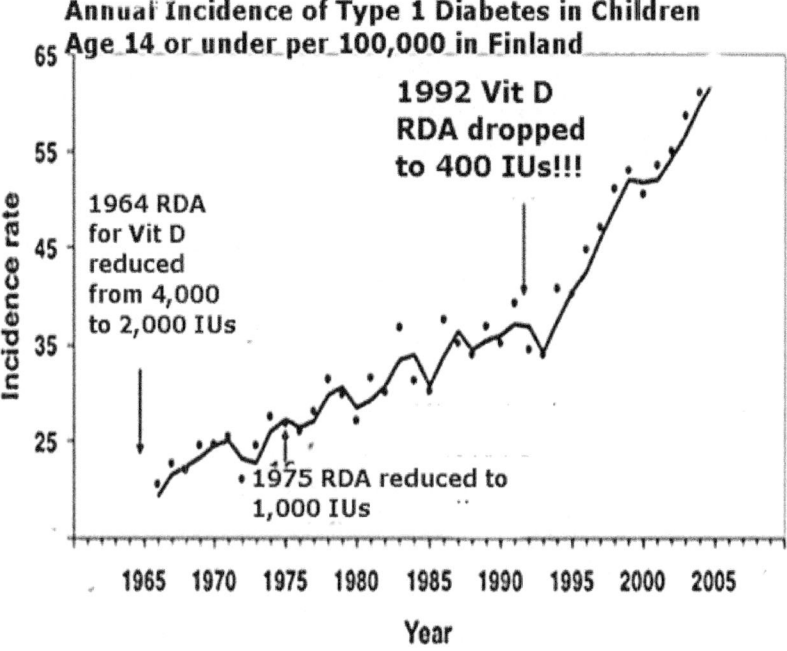

3. Rheumatoid Arthritis:
   - While data varies, some regions report up to a 2.5% annual increase since the 1980s.
4. Inflammatory Bowel Disease (IBD):
   - Both Crohn's disease and ulcerative colitis show increased incidence.
   - Some studies report a doubling of cases over the past three decades.

Cancer
1. Breast Cancer:
   - Incidence rates have increased by about 30% since the 1980s in many developed countries.

2. Prostate Cancer:
   - Sharp increase in diagnosed cases.
3. Colorectal Cancer:
   - While overall rates have decreased in older adults due to screening, there's been an alarming increase in young adults.
4. Thyroid cancer has exploded by 1,000's of percent!
5.

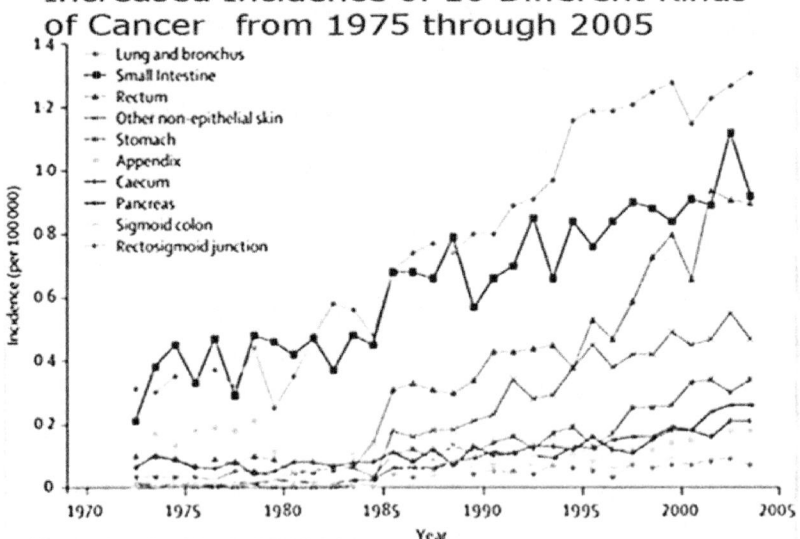

Metabolic Disorders
1. Type 2 Diabetes:

- Dramatic increase, with some countries reporting a doubling or tripling of cases since the 1980s.
2. Obesity:
    - Rates have skyrocketed in many countries since 1980.
    - Childhood obesity has become a particular concern.

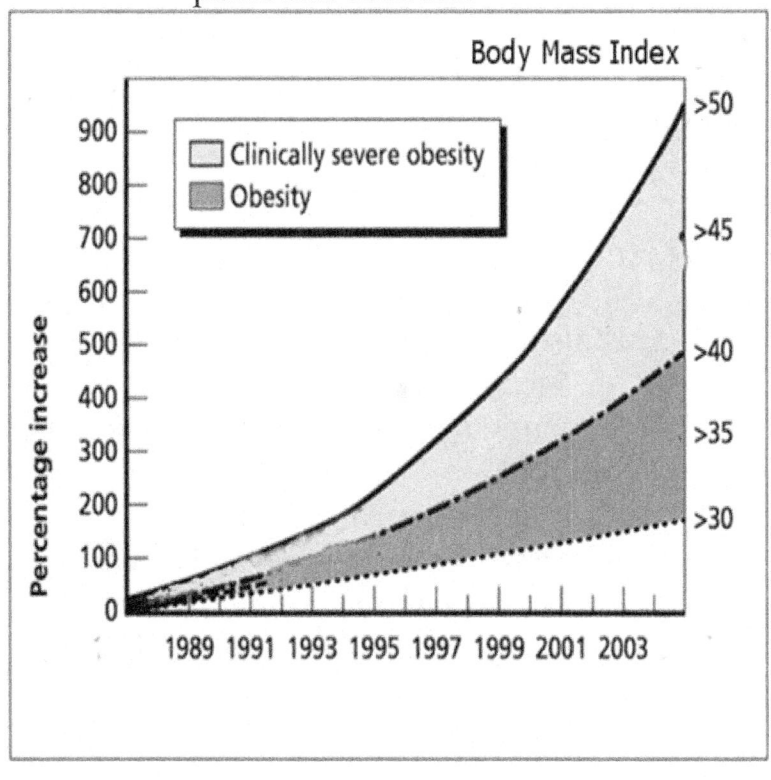

Cardiovascular Diseases
1. Hypertension:
   - Significant increase in prevalence, especially in developing countries.

2. Heart Failure:
   - While mortality has decreased due to better treatments, incidence has increased.

Neurological Disorders
1. Alzheimer's Disease:
   - Incidence has risen sharply, with some estimates suggesting a doubling every 20 years.
2. Parkinson's Disease:
   - Steady increase in incidence, particularly in industrialized nations.

Other Conditions
1. Autism Spectrum Disorders:
   - Dramatic increase in autism cases diagnosed. (One study found that supplementing expectant mothers with 6000 Ius of D3 per day completely eliminated autistic births in women who had prior autistic births).

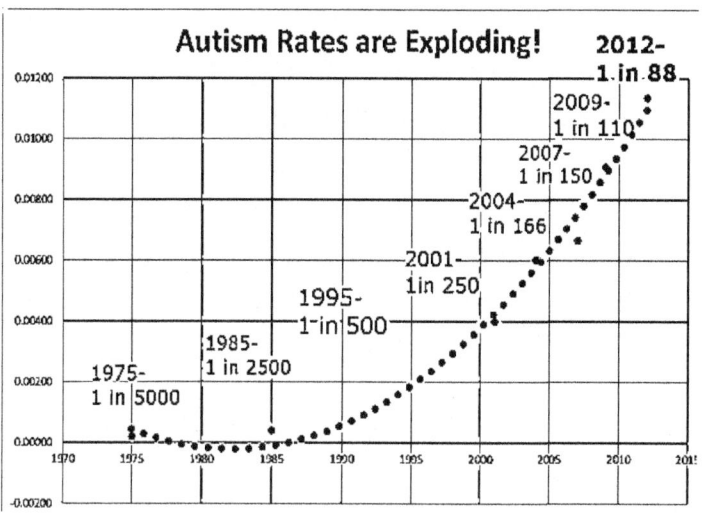

2. Allergies and Asthma:
    - Significant increase in prevalence, especially in children.
3. Depression and Anxiety Disorders:
    - Marked increase in diagnosed cases across all age groups.

This widespread increase in various diseases and conditions correlates strongly with the promotion of sun avoidance and sunscreen use beginning in the 1980s. The resulting vitamin D deficiency is the main contributing factor to these trends.

Remarkable Results of High-Dose Vitamin D3 Supplementation

High-dose vitamin D3 supplementation has shown extraordinary results in treating various health conditions. Here's a summary of some of the most notable findings:

Autoimmune Diseases: The Coimbra Protocol

Dr. Cicero Coimbra, a neurologist from Brazil, has developed a protocol using high-dose vitamin D3 (1,000 IUs of D3 per kg of body weight per day) to treat autoimmune diseases with remarkable success:
- Multiple Sclerosis (MS): Many patients have experienced complete remission of symptoms, with some regaining the ability to walk after being wheelchair-bound.
- Psoriasis: Patients have reported significant improvement or complete clearing of skin lesions.
- Vitiligo: Cases of repigmentation have been observed in patients following the protocol.
- Rheumatoid Arthritis: Substantial reduction in joint pain and inflammation has been reported.

- Crohn's Disease: Patients have experienced remission of symptoms and improved quality of life.
- Many more autoimmune and other diseases have also been cured with this protocol including acne, depression, lupus, asthma, myasthenia gravis, etc.

The Coimbra Protocol typically involves:

- Daily doses of vitamin D3 ranging from 10,000 IU to 300,000 IU or more, tailored to each patient. (His general approach is 1,000 IUs of D3 per kg of body weight per day).
- Regular monitoring of calcium levels in blood and urine.
- Dietary restrictions to limit calcium intake.
- Supplementation with magnesium to support proper calcium metabolism.
- Unfortunately, Coimbra does not recommend vitamin K2 and thus his calcium dietary restrictions have led most of his adherents to suffer from decreased bone density. I believe he made this mistake because when he tested his patients who took vitamin K2 he saw an initial increase in blood calcium. If the K2 was acting to decalcify soft tissues this would be expected as the calcium has to

pass through the blood to get back into the bones. Adding K2 to his regimen would likely lower blood calcium levels in the longer run and allow his patients to drop the calcium intake restrictions and prevent the loss of their BMD.

Cancer Prevention and Treatment

While not yet thought of as a cure by most, high-dose vitamin D3 has shown potential in cancer prevention and as an adjunct to conventional treatments:

- Breast Cancer: Studies have shown that women with higher vitamin D levels have a lower risk of developing breast cancer.
- Colorectal Cancer: Higher vitamin D levels are associated with reduced risk and improved survival rates.
- Prostate Cancer: Some studies suggest that vitamin D may slow the progression of prostate cancer.
- The author has heard form quite a few high dose D3 experimenters that claim their cancers were put into complete remission after taking high dose D3 (10,000 to 50,000 Ius per day including several cases of prostate cancer).

Cardiovascular Health

High-dose vitamin D3 supplementation has been linked to improvements in cardiovascular health:
- Blood Pressure: Some patients have reported normalization of blood pressure after starting high-dose vitamin D3 therapy.
- Cholesterol Levels: Improvements in lipid profiles have been observed in some individuals.

Neurological Conditions
Beyond MS, high-dose vitamin D3 has shown promise in other neurological conditions:
- Parkinson's Disease: Some patients have reported improved motor function and reduced tremors.
- Alzheimer's Disease: Preliminary research suggests that vitamin D may play a role in cognitive function and neuroprotection.

Metabolic Health
High-dose vitamin D3 supplementation has been associated with improvements in metabolic health:

- Type 2 Diabetes: Some studies suggest that vitamin D may improve insulin sensitivity and glucose metabolism.
- Obesity: Higher vitamin D levels have been linked to improved weight management in some individuals. In my book "Why are there no fat people in Colorado?" the case is made that the obesity map of the US can be completely explained by the varying levels of vitamin D3 in the population where populations with a high percentage of dark pigmented people were found to be obese. Other pockets of obesity on the map include white people in the Appalacian mountains (low altitude shadow-inducing mountains that reduce the amount of sunlight received each day). Elderly people in New England because elderly skin does not make as much D3 as young skin (less than 50%).

And then there are the people of Colorado live in mountain shadows as well, who should be fat but generally are not. It turns out that the higher altitude / thin air allows much more intense UVB radiation (up to 70% stronger than at sea level) to get through thus more than offsetting the increase in shadows from the mountains.

In fact, the book about Colorado just mentioned was originally titled "16 fascinating Covid and Spanish Flu mysteries Solved" which was banned by Amazon for 3 years. It turns out that variations in vitamin D3 levels which can explain the US obesity map can also explain the US Covid map.

Immune Function and Infection Resistance

Vitamin D plays a crucial role in immune function:
- Respiratory Infections: Higher vitamin D levels have been associated with reduced risk and severity of respiratory infections, including influenza and COVID-19.
- Studies have shown that vitamin d3 supplementation is up to 10x more effective than the flu vaccines at preventing the flu in vitamin D3 deficient people.
- Since taking a minimum of 4000 IUs of vitamin D3 per day I personally have only had a single cold in the last 25 years during a D3 wash out period.
- At the first sign of a cold, some vitamin D3 researchers advocate that taking 50,000 IUs of vitamin D3 for 3 days in a row or

more will usually knock it out before it takes hold.
- Autoimmune Regulation: Vitamin D helps modulate the immune system, potentially preventing the acquisition of autoimmune disorders.

Mental Health

Some patients have reported improvements in mental health conditions with high-dose vitamin D3 supplementation:
- Depression: Vitamin D deficiency has been linked to depression, and some individuals have reported dramatic mood improvements with supplementation with some getting rid of their Prozac which they claim makes them feel numb while the high dose D3 (30,000 Ius/day +) makes them feel alive and full of energy.
- Anxiety: Anecdotal reports suggest potential benefits for anxiety symptoms. (However, magnesium seems the best for this as one symptom of magnesium deficiency is anxiety and another panic attacks)
- Because schizophrenia and bipolar disorder both show a latitude effect like other diseases, vitamin D3 may prevent

these diseases and may even help treat them.

Safety and Monitoring

While high-dose vitamin D3 therapy has shown promising results, it's crucial to note:
- The importance of medical supervision and regular monitoring of blood calcium levels and kidney function. (Actually, I have heard from a number of people that high dose D3 completely reversed their chronic kidney failure).
- The need for adequate hydration and dietary calcium restriction to prevent hypercalcemia. (Or make sure you are taking adequate vitamin K2 to prevent hypercalcemia).
- The role of cofactors like magnesium and vitamin K2 in supporting proper vitamin D metabolism and preventing potential side effects.

These findings highlight the potential of high-dose vitamin D3 as a powerful tool in managing various health conditions.

Remarkable Results of High-Dose Vitamin D3 Supplementation

Anecdotal Cancer Cases

While anecdotal evidence should be interpreted cautiously, some remarkable cases have been reported:

Ovarian Cancer Case
A woman diagnosed with stage 4 ovarian cancer opted for high-dose vitamin D3 therapy:
- She took 50,000 IU of vitamin D3 daily.
- After several months, her cancer markers dropped significantly.
- Subsequent scans showed no evidence of cancer.
- She continued the high-dose regimen and remained cancer-free for years.

Pancreatic Cancer in an Elderly Patient
An elderly woman diagnosed with pancreatic cancer, typically associated with poor prognosis, experienced an unexpected outcome:
- She began accidentally taking 50,000 IU of vitamin D3 daily. (Instead of 5,000 IUs as recommended by her holistic health coach).
- Doctor's put her on chemotherapy designed to extend her life about 5 months.

After a bad reaction to the first chemo treatment, she was considered unable to continue with it and was sent home to die.
- Despite the aggressive nature of pancreatic cancer, her condition stabilized.
- The doctors were shocked when they checked on her about a year later to find out she was still alive and claimed to have never felt better in her life!
- X rays showed her pancreatic tumor had actually shrunk somewhat.
- Her case was written up and published with the title "The Incidental Use of High-Dose Vitamin D3 in Pancreatic Cancer".

Prostate Cancer Research by Dr. Bruce Hollis

After significant obstacles in getting approval for "such a dangerously high dose of D3" from government regulators, Dr. Bruce Hollis's research on vitamin D3 supplementation in prostate cancer patients yielded significant findings:
- Study Design: Men with low-risk prostate cancer were given 4,000 IU of vitamin D3 daily for a year before their scheduled prostatectomy.
- Results:
    - Patients taking vitamin D3 had significantly fewer tumors compared to the control group.

- The tumors found in the vitamin D3 group were notably smaller.
- Some patients in the vitamin D3 group showed no evidence of cancer at the time of surgery.
- Implications: These findings suggest that vitamin D3 supplementation may play a role in slowing or potentially reversing the progression of early-stage prostate cancer.
- Dr. Hollis stated that if he ever got prostate cancer, he would probably take 50,000 IUs a day.
- He claims that the prestigious medical journals would not touch his study and he had to publish it in an obscure journal.

These cases and research findings, while not definitive proof, add to the growing body of evidence suggesting the potential benefits of high-dose vitamin D3 supplementation in cancer prevention and treatment. They underscore the need for further rigorous clinical trials to fully understand the role of vitamin D3 in cancer management.

Vitamin D3 may play a crucial role in combating cancer by enhancing mitochondrial function, which aligns with Dr. Thomas Seyfried's metabolic theory of cancer. This theory posits that cancer is primarily a mitochondrial metabolic disease rather than a genetic one. As proof, he has shown that mitochondrial transplants to replace faulty mitochondria have resulted in the normalization of cancer cells into normal cells. He has also noted that cancerous embryonic stem cells when fused with cells with normal mitochondria can often develop into perfectly normal organisms.

Here's a summary of how vitamin D3 might help kill cancer cells through mitochondrial enhancement:

Vitamin D3 and Mitochondrial Function

In addition to revving up the immune system to kill off the bad actors like nascent cancer cells and bacterial, fungal and viral infections, research has shown that vitamin D3, particularly its active form 1,25(OH)2D3, can significantly improve mitochondrial function:

- In skeletal muscle cells, vitamin D3 supplementation increases mitochondrial respiration rates and ATP production
- Treatment with 1,25(OH)2D3 enhances mitochondrial complex I-IV activities and citrate synthase activity in both mouse and human muscle cells

- Vitamin D3 therapy has been associated with improved maximal oxidative phosphorylation in human subjects with vitamin D deficiency

Connection to Seyfried's Metabolic Theory

Dr. Seyfried's theory suggests that cancer arises from chronic mitochondrial damage and compensatory fermentation. This aligns with the potential anti-cancer effects of vitamin D3:

- By enhancing mitochondrial function, vitamin D3 may help restore normal cellular respiration in cancer cells.
- Improved mitochondrial function could potentially reverse the Warburg effect, where cancer cells rely heavily on glucose fermentation for energy.
- Enhanced mitochondrial activity might reactivate apoptosis pathways in cancer cells, promoting their death.

Potential Mechanisms
1. Gene Expression: Vitamin D3 modulates the expression of genes involved in mitochondrial biogenesis and function.
2. Metabolic Reprogramming: 1,25(OH)2D3 has been shown to influence metabolic pathways in cancer cells, potentially

shifting them away from the fermentative metabolism that supports their growth.
3. Autophagy Regulation: Vitamin D3 can induce autophagy in cancer cells, which may help eliminate dysfunctional mitochondria and promote cellular health.
4. AMPK Activation: 1,25(OH)2D3 activates AMPK, an energy sensor that can regulate metabolism and potentially inhibit cancer cell growth.

Implications for Cancer Treatment

The potential of vitamin D3 to enhance mitochondrial function in cancer cells could have significant implications for treatment:
- It may sensitize cancer cells to other therapies by improving their metabolic health.
- Combining vitamin D3 with metabolic therapies, such as the ketogenic diet suggested by Seyfried, might synergistically target cancer's metabolic vulnerabilities.
- Vitamin D3 supplementation could potentially be used as a preventive measure against cancer by maintaining healthy mitochondrial function.

- It is my and others' observations that curing autoimmune diseases, triggering the tissue remodeling program require vitamin D3 blood levels of 125 ng/ml or higher, and this likely applies to optimal cancer therapy using vitamin D3.

While these findings are promising, it's important to note that more research is needed to fully understand the therapeutic potential of vitamin D3 in cancer treatment. The approach of targeting cancer's metabolic abnormalities, as suggested by both vitamin D3 research and Seyfried's theory, represents an exciting avenue for future cancer therapies.

The COVID-19 Pandemic and Vitamin D3

Higher vitamin D3 levels in the population could have potentially prevented or significantly mitigated the COVID-19 pandemic:
1. Enhanced Immune Function:
    - Vitamin D3 plays a crucial role in modulating the immune system, enhancing innate immunity while regulating excessive inflammatory responses.
    - Adequate vitamin D levels could have improved the population's

overall resistance to SARS-CoV-2 infection.
2. Reduced Severity of Infections:
    - Studies show that individuals with higher vitamin D levels experienced less severe COVID-19 symptoms and had lower hospitalization rates.
    - Vitamin D deficiency was associated with increased risk of ICU admission and mortality in COVID-19 patients.
3. Prevention of Cytokine Storms:
    - Vitamin D3 helps regulate the production of inflammatory cytokines.
    - Adequate levels could have prevented the dangerous cytokine storms observed in severe COVID-19 cases.
4. Improved Respiratory Function:
    - Vitamin D3 plays a role in maintaining healthy lung tissue and function.
    - Higher vitamin D3 levels are associated with better outcomes in respiratory infections, including those caused by coronaviruses.
5. Population-wide Protection:
    - If the general population had maintained vitamin D levels above

50 ng/mL through supplementation (typically requiring 5,000-10,000 IU daily for adults), the spread and severity of COVID-19 could have been dramatically reduced or completely avoided.

6. Cost-effective Prevention:
   - Vitamin D3 supplementation is inexpensive compared to the economic costs of lockdowns and medical treatments.
   - Widespread vitamin D3 supplementation could have been a cost-effective strategy to mitigate the pandemic.
7. Reduced Comorbidity Risks:
   - Many conditions associated with severe COVID-19 outcomes (obesity, diabetes, hypertension) are also linked to vitamin D deficiency.

Suppression of Vitamin D3 Information

The CDC, NIH, and other major health institutions have downplayed and /or dismissed the importance of vitamin D3 in combating COVID-19, despite growing evidence of its effectiveness. When I was researching their websites to get Covid information in 2021-2022,

I found nothing but disinformation: Key points include:

1. Ignoring or Downplaying Studies: The CDC and NIH have reportedly ignored or minimized the results of numerous studies showing a strong correlation between vitamin D levels and COVID-19 outcomes
2. Lack of Promotion: Despite low-cost and low-risk nature of vitamin D supplementation, these agencies have not promoted it as a potential preventive measure against COVID-19.
3. Emphasis on Vaccines: There has been an overemphasis on vaccine development and distribution, while potentially effective and immediately available interventions like vitamin D supplementation were sidelined.
4. Conflicts of Interest: Financial interests in vaccine development and other pharmaceutical interventions likely were influencing the agencies' stance on vitamin D.
5. Inconsistent Messaging: While acknowledging vitamin D's importance for overall health, the CDC and NIH have been reluctant to recommend it specifically for COVID-19 prevention or treatment. And they still recommend the completely

ineffective doses of 600 to 800 IUs per day as promoted by the IOM.

False Information

These agencies provided misleading or false information in several ways:
1. Claiming Lack of Evidence: The CDC and NIH on their websites have stated that there is insufficient evidence to recommend vitamin D for COVID-19, despite numerous studies suggesting otherwise.
2. Downplaying Effectiveness: When mentioning vitamin D, these agencies often emphasize its general health benefits rather than its potential specific role in fighting COVID-19.
3. Overemphasis on Potential Risks: The agencies exaggerate the risks of vitamin D toxicity while understating its benefits in the context of the pandemic.
4. Selective Citation of Studies: These agencies are selectively citing studies that do not show strong benefits of vitamin D, while ignoring those that do.

This suppression and misinformation may have cost thousands if not millions of lives by preventing the widespread adoption of a simple, low-cost intervention that could have significantly impacted the course of the pandemic.

There is evidence suggesting that the CDC and NIH have misrepresented or downplayed research on vitamin D3's potential role in combating COVID-19. Here is a detailed example of how one study was allegedly misinterpreted:

Misinterpretation of Vitamin D3 Study

A key instance of misrepresentation involves a study published in JAMA Network Open in September 2020
This study, conducted by researchers at the University of Chicago Medicine, examined the relationship between vitamin D levels and COVID-19 risk.
The Study's Actual Findings
The research found that patients with vitamin D deficiency (defined as less than 20 ng/mL) were 77% more likely to test positive for COVID-19 compared to patients with sufficient vitamin D levels. This suggested a strong correlation between vitamin D status and COVID-19 susceptibility.

CDC/NIH Misrepresentation

However, when referencing this study, the CDC and NIH:
1. Downplayed the significance of the findings by emphasizing that the study was observational and could not prove causation.
2. Focused on the limitations section of the study, highlighting potential confounding factors while minimizing the strong association found.
3. Used language that suggested the results were inconclusive, despite the clear statistical significance of the findings.
4. Omitted mentioning the 77% increased risk figure in their public communications about vitamin D and COVID-19.
5. Concluded that there was "insufficient evidence" to recommend vitamin D for COVID-19 prevention or treatment, despite this study and others suggesting a potential benefit.

Implications

By misrepresenting the study's findings, the CDC and NIH effectively reversed the study's implications. Instead of acknowledging the potential importance of vitamin D status in

COVID-19 risk, they used the study to justify their position that vitamin D supplementation was not recommended for COVID-19. This misinterpretation may have discouraged further research into vitamin D's role in COVID-19 and potentially deprived the public of a low-cost, low-risk intervention that could have reduced disease severity and mortality rates.

The NIH has also on its website misrepresented or downplayed the results of studies examining the relationship between vitamin D and COVID-19 outcomes. Here's a summary of the key points:

1. The NIH claimed "clear evidence that vitamin D supplementation provides protection against infection or improves outcomes in patients with COVID-19 is still lacking," despite multiple observational studies suggesting otherwise.
2. In a study of healthcare workers, the NIH downplayed significant results showing that only 6.4% of participants in the vitamin D3 group acquired SARS-CoV-2 infection compared to 24.5% in the placebo group.
3. The NIH cited studies using large single doses of inactive vitamin D3 in severely ill patients, which showed no effect, without acknowledging the potential issues with this approach.

4. Most egregiously, the NIH misrepresented the results of a study using calcitriol (the most active form of vitamin D3) in hospitalized COVID-19 patients:
    - They acknowledged a statistically significant improvement in oxygenation but failed to emphasize the magnitude of the improvement (a 91.04 vs 13.2- increase in the SaO2/FiO2 ratio).
    - The NIH claimed "There were no differences between the arms in the length of hospital stay, mortality, or the need for ICU admission or hospital readmission." However, the actual study results showed:
        - Average length of stay: 5.5 days (calcitriol) vs 9.24 days (control)
        - ICU transfers: 5 (calcitriol) vs 8 (control)
        - Deaths: 0 (calcitriol) vs 3 (control)
        - Readmissions: 2 (calcitriol) vs 4 (control)

This misrepresentation of study results on the NIH website appears to be a deliberate attempt to downplay the potential benefits of vitamin D in COVID-19 prevention and treatment. Such actions raise serious concerns about the accuracy and objectivity of information provided by public health institutions.

Large amounts of vitamin D misinformation that continues to remain on the NIH and CDC's websites as of 11/2024.

Critique of Current Research

The VITAL Study: A Flawed Approach to Vitamin D3 Research

The VITAL (VITamin D and OmegA-3 TriaL) study, while widely publicized, represents a problematic approach to investigating the benefits of vitamin D3 supplementation. Despite its large scale and lengthy duration, the study's design and interpretation raise significant concerns about its validity and the conclusions drawn from its results.

Inadequate Dosage: Setting the Stage for Failure

The VITAL study's fundamental flaw lies in its choice of vitamin D3 dosage. By administering only 2,000 IU per day, the researchers selected a dose that many experts consider insufficient to produce meaningful health benefits. This dosage is far below the levels that the human body can naturally produce when exposed to adequate sunlight. To put this in perspective:

- The human body can produce up to 20,000 IU of vitamin D3 in just 15-30 minutes of full-body sun exposure. Thus 2,000 IUs represents the amount one could make from sunbathing for just 1.5 to 3 minutes per day!
- Many vitamin D researchers recommend daily intakes of around 10,000 IU for optimal health benefits.
- The 2,000 IU dose used in VITAL is barely enough to raise serum 25(OH)D levels above the minimum threshold considered necessary for basic health maintenance.

By choosing such a conservative dose, the VITAL study essentially set itself up to find minimal or no effects. This approach ignores the growing body of research suggesting that higher doses are necessary to achieve optimal vitamin D status and realize its full health potential.

Baseline Vitamin D Levels: A Critical Oversight

Another significant issue with the VITAL study is its failure to adequately account for participants' baseline vitamin D levels. The study reported that participants had a mean baseline 25(OH)D concentration of 30.8 ng/mL, which is already at the lower end of what many "experts" consider sufficient. This presents several problems:

1. Participants were not vitamin D deficient at baseline, limiting the potential for improvement.
2. The small increase in serum levels achieved by supplementation (to 41.2 ng/mL) may not have been sufficient to demonstrate significant health benefits.
3. The study did not stratify results based on baseline vitamin D status, potentially masking benefits in truly deficient individuals.

Misinterpretation of Results: Ignoring Positive Findings

While the VITAL study's primary endpoints showed no significant benefits for cardiovascular disease or cancer prevention, it's crucial to note

that several secondary analyses did reveal positive outcomes:
1. A 22% reduction in autoimmune disease incidence was observed in the vitamin D group.
2. There was a significant reduction in cancer mortality (not incidence) in the vitamin D group, particularly after excluding the first two years of follow-up.
3. Subgroup analyses suggested benefits for certain populations, such as those with lower BMI or lower baseline fish oil intake.

Despite these promising findings, many interpretations of the VITAL study have focused solely on the primary endpoints, leading to overly broad conclusions about vitamin D's ineffectiveness.

The Potential for Disinformation

The way the VITAL study has been presented and interpreted raises concerns about potential conflicts of interest and the influence of pharmaceutical industry interests. By promoting a narrative that vitamin D supplementation is unnecessary, several parties stand to benefit:

1. Pharmaceutical companies producing medications for conditions that vitamin D might help prevent or treat.
2. Sunscreen manufacturers and dermatology groups advocating for minimal sun exposure.
3. Food industry players who benefit from the continued focus on calcium rather than vitamin D for bone health.

It's important to consider these potential conflicts when evaluating the study's conclusions and their widespread promotion in medical and public health circles.

Overlooking Cofactors: The Magnesium Connection

The VITAL study, like many vitamin D trials, failed to adequately address the crucial role of magnesium in vitamin D metabolism. Magnesium is essential for the activation of vitamin D, and deficiency in this mineral can limit the effectiveness of vitamin D supplementation. Recent research has shown that:

- Up to 80% of Americans may be magnesium deficient.

- Magnesium is required for the conversion of vitamin D into its active form.
- Without sufficient magnesium, vitamin D may remain stored and inactive.

By not accounting for participants' magnesium status or ensuring adequate magnesium intake, the VITAL study may have underestimated the potential benefits of vitamin D supplementation.

The Latitude Effect: A Missed Opportunity

One of the most compelling arguments for the importance of vitamin D comes from epidemiological studies showing the "latitude effect" in cancer rates and other diseases. People living closer to the equator, where sun exposure and vitamin D production are higher, tend to have dramatically lower rates of many cancers, autoimmune, and other diseases and conditions. The VITAL study, conducted primarily in the United States, did not adequately explore this geographical variation. By failing to stratify results based on latitude or baseline sun exposure, the study missed an opportunity to investigate how vitamin D supplementation might differentially benefit populations with varying natural vitamin D production.

Beyond Bone Health: Vitamin D's Multifaceted Role

While the VITAL study focused primarily on cardiovascular disease and cancer, it's crucial to recognize vitamin D's wide-ranging effects on human health. Vitamin D receptors are found in nearly every cell in the body, suggesting a role far beyond bone metabolism. Areas where vitamin D shows huge promise include:

1. Immune function and autoimmune disease prevention
2. Neurological health and cognitive function
3. Muscle strength and fall prevention (with sufficient magnesium co-supplementation)
4. Respiratory health, including protection against infections
5. Metabolic health and diabetes prevention

By narrowly focusing on specific endpoints, the VITAL study may have overlooked significant benefits in other areas of health.

The Need for Personalized Approaches

One of the most significant shortcomings of large-scale studies like VITAL is their inability to account for individual variations in vitamin D metabolism and requirements. Factors that can

influence an individual's vitamin D needs include:
- Skin pigmentation (melanin is basically the body's version of sun block)
- Age
- Body mass index
- Genetic variations in vitamin D receptors and metabolizing enzymes
- Concurrent health conditions
- Medication use

A one-dose-fits-all approach to vitamin D supplementation, as used in the VITAL study, fails to address these crucial individual differences. At a minimum blood levels of D3 should have been measured and targeted with much more blood testing rather than selecting a one dose fits all approach.

The conflicting results from various studies highlight the need for a more nuanced approach to vitamin D3 supplementation. Factors such as baseline vitamin D status, body mass index, age, and overall health status can all influence an individual's response to supplementation. People respond differently to the same dose of vitamin D3 so it is essential that one gets one's blood tested during a high dose vitamin D3 regimen. While the "normal" reference range in the US is 30 to 100 ng/ml (or 75 to 250 nmol/L); it is the author's and others' experience that cures for autoimmune diseases and the triggering of the tissue remodeling system does not occur at blood levels under 125 ng/ml. In fact, I know of one lady who cured her Crohn's disease of 50 years only when her D3 blood levels were 150 ng/ml or above. It would come back if she let the level drop to the 100 to 120 ng/ml range.

A personalized approach to supplementation could help maximize the benefits of vitamin D3 while minimizing potential risks.

Reinterpreting VITAL: A Call for Nuanced Analysis

Rather than dismissing vitamin D supplementation based on VITAL's primary outcomes, a more nuanced interpretation of the study is warranted:
1. The reduction in (and cure of) autoimmune diseases suggests significant potential benefits, particularly given the rising prevalence of these conditions.
2. The observed reduction in cancer mortality, while not meeting the primary endpoint criteria, is clinically significant and deserves further investigation.

3. Subgroup analyses indicating benefits for certain populations highlight the need for targeted supplementation strategies.
4. The study's limitations, including dosage and baseline vitamin D status, should be clearly acknowledged when interpreting results.

Moving Forward: Recommendations for Future Research

Recently the large-scale (25,000+ participants) VITAL trial has failed to provide any valuable insights into the effects of vitamin D3 supplementation, and in effect is basically, I believe, just disinformation meant to discredit the health benefits of vitamin D3.

By using such a low dose of vitamin D3 (2000 IUs or the sunbathing equivalent of 3 minutes per day)- this study was designed to fail.

The shocking ignorance surrounding vitamin D3 has had far-reaching consequences on public health. By addressing this knowledge gap and correcting longstanding errors, we can potentially revolutionize our approach to preventing and treating a wide range of diseases, from autoimmune disorders to cancer and infectious diseases like COVID-19.

Unfortunately, the emerging evidence from large-scale junk science trials like VITAL (designed to fail) provides a platform from which Big Pharma and its shills can discredit the benefits of vitamin D3.

To address the shortcomings of the VITAL study and advance our understanding of vitamin D's health impacts, future research should consider:

1. Testing higher doses of vitamin D3, minimally using 10,000 IU per day and using doses as high as 50,000 a day or even higher.
2. Stratifying participants based on baseline vitamin D status and targeting those with true deficiency.
3. Incorporating measures of magnesium status and ensuring adequate magnesium intake.
4. Incorporating measures of vitamin K2 status and ensuring adequate vitamin K2 magnesium intake.
5. Investigating the effects of vitamin D supplementation across different latitudes and in populations with varying sun exposure.
6. Utilizing more sensitive markers of vitamin D status beyond serum 25(OH)D, such as the vitamin D metabolome.
7. Long-term effects: Most studies have followed participants for 3-5 years. Longer-term studies could reveal additional benefits or risks associated with sustained vitamin D3 supplementation.

8. Genetic factors: Investigating how genetic variations influence vitamin D metabolism and response to supplementation could help tailor recommendations to individual needs as some people suffer from vitamin D3 receptor polymorphisms that make them more resistant to the effects vitamin D3.
9. Combination therapies: Further studies on the synergistic effects of vitamin D3 with other nutrients, such as magnesium and vitamin K2, (and boron, zinc, and vitamin A) could lead to more effective supplementation strategies that allow for much higher doses.
10. Younger populations: Most large-scale trials have focused on older adults. Investigating the effects of vitamin D3 supplementation in younger age groups could provide insights into its potential for disease prevention earlier in life. Also, as one ages the function of Vitamin D3 receptors declines requiring even higher doses in the elderly to achieve the same results that occur in younger people with smaller doses

The Vital Study Did Hint at Some Positive Benefits

for Such a Small Dose of D3 (2000 IUs = the equivalent of a light skinned person sunbathing for 1.5 to 3 minutes a day):

Autoimmune Diseases

The VITAL study, a randomized double-blind placebo-controlled trial following more than 25,000 men and women ages 50 and older, found that taking vitamin D supplements (2,000 IU/day) for five years reduced the incidence of autoimmune diseases by about 22%, compared with a placebo. Autoimmune conditions observed included rheumatoid arthritis, psoriasis, polymyalgia rheumatica, and autoimmune thyroid diseases (Hashimoto's thyroiditis, Graves' disease, and more).

Dr. Karen Costenbader of the Brigham's Division of Rheumatology, Inflammation and Immunity stated, "This is the first direct evidence we have that daily supplementation may reduce autoimmune disease incidence, and what looks like more pronounced effect after two years of supplementation for vitamin D."

Cancer Prevention and Mortality

While the VITAL study did not show a significant reduction in overall cancer incidence with vitamin D3 supplementation, it did reveal some promising results:
1. A secondary analysis of the VITAL trial found that vitamin D3 supplementation reduced the incidence of advanced (metastatic or fatal) cancer in the overall cohort, with the strongest risk reduction observed in individuals with normal weight (larger people need larger doses of D3).
2. A meta-analysis of 10 randomized controlled trials through 2018 (including the VITAL trial) found that vitamin D supplementation was associated with a slight (13%) reduction in cancer mortality over 3–10 years of follow-up.

These findings suggest that vitamin D3 plays a role in reducing cancer progression and mortality, even at very small doses.

Practical Implications: What This Means for Public Health

Despite the limitations of the VITAL study, it's crucial not to dismiss the potential benefits of

vitamin D supplementation. Instead, a more nuanced approach to public health recommendations is needed:
1. Encourage regular testing of vitamin D levels, particularly for individuals at high risk of deficiency.
2. Promote safe sun exposure as a natural way to boost vitamin D levels, while being mindful of skin cancer risks.
3. Recognize that optimal vitamin D levels may vary based on individual factors and health goals.
4. Consider higher supplementation doses for individuals with documented deficiency or specific health concerns.
5. Emphasize the importance of magnesium and other cofactors in vitamin D metabolism.
6. Educate healthcare providers on the complexities of vitamin D metabolism and the limitations of current research.

A Call for Critical Thinking

The VITAL study, has significantly influenced public health policy and medical practice regarding vitamin D supplementation.

According to Dr. Bruce Hollis -

the VITAL study has effectively made it impossible to get funding for any further research on vitamin D3.

It is also being used by apparent shills for Big Pharma to discourage the use of taking vitamin D3 by the general population. Consider the editorial by Clifford Rosen an editor for The New England Journal of Medicine about the VITAL study being run by Joanne Manson of Harvard.

(It is interesting to note that both Clifford Rosen and Joanne Manson were members of the IOM committee (Institute of Medicine) when they made the decimal point error in their recommendation for the daily dose of vitamin D3 of a criminally low 600 to 800 IUs per day instead of 6000 to 8000 a day as calculated by the 2 groups of researchers who checked their work!

Summary of Dr. Clifford Rosen's Editorial About the VITAL Study

Context

Dr. Rosen's editorial was published alongside the results of the VITAL study in the New England Journal of Medicine.

Main Arguments
1. Lack of Benefit: Dr. Rosen emphasizes that the VITAL study found no significant reduction in cancer or cardiovascular events with vitamin D supplementation.
2. Questioning Previous Observational Studies: He suggests that the results challenge the findings of numerous observational studies that had previously linked low vitamin D levels to various diseases.
3. Dosage Considerations: Rosen notes that the dose used in VITAL (2000 IU daily) was higher than in previous trials. (Which means all the stuffies using even lower doses were also a waste of time and money).
4. Baseline Vitamin D Levels: He points out that participants' baseline vitamin D levels were relatively high, which could have

limited the potential benefits of supplementation.
5. Subgroup Analyses: Rosen acknowledges some positive findings in subgroup analyses, such as a possible reduction in cancer deaths after excluding the first two years of the trial.
6. Implications for Clinical Practice: Despite these subgroup findings, Rosen argues that they do not justify widespread vitamin D supplementation for cancer or cardiovascular disease prevention.
7. Future Research: He suggests that future studies should focus on populations with clear vitamin D deficiency or those at high risk for specific outcomes.

Rosen's Conclusion

Dr. Rosen concludes that the VITAL results do not support the use of vitamin D supplements for preventing cancer or cardiovascular disease in the general population!

He suggests that the era of vitamin D as a panacea for chronic disease prevention may be over.

Why the hostility? Consider this:

Biologics: A Double-Edged Sword

Modern biologic drugs for autoimmune conditions and cancers operate by targeting specific parts of the immune system. However, this targeted approach comes with significant drawbacks:
- Autoimmune disease biologics suppress parts of the immune system, leading to increased risk of infections and cancers as side effects.
- Cancer biologics rev up certain immune responses, but can trigger autoimmune diseases as a side effect.

For example, the cancer drug Keytruda can cause immune-mediated pneumonitis, colitis, hepatitis and other autoimmune reactions. Meanwhile, the autoimmune drug Humira carries risks of serious infections and lymphoma.

The Price of Precision

These biologics come at an enormous cost:
- Ocrelizumab for MS: $65,000 per year
- Many other biologics: Tens of thousands of dollars annually

The Ultimate Biologic: Vitamin D3

In contrast, vitamin D3 acts as a master regulator of the entire immune system:
- Fine-tunes immune responses across the board
- Helps prevent both autoimmune diseases and cancers
- Has virtually no side effects when used properly
- Costs as little as $50 per year

The MS Example: David vs. Goliath

The case of multiple sclerosis (MS) treatment illustrates the stark contrast between Big Pharma biologics and vitamin D3:
- New MS drug ocrelizumab: $65,000/year, slows disease progression by 24%
- High-dose vitamin D3 therapy: $50/year, halts or eliminates MS in up to 95% of cases

Dr. Cicero Coimbra in Brazil has successfully treated over 5,000 MS patients using high-dose vitamin D3, with a claimed 95% success rate. Patients around the world are now curing their MS using this approach, as evidenced by numerous testimonials and Facebook support groups.

The Hostility of Big Medicine

Despite its promise, the medical establishment remains hostile to high-dose vitamin D3 therapy:
- It is claimed that the overbuilt for-profit hospitals were nearly empty in the 1920s-30s when people began taking high doses of the newly discovered vitamin D.
- Medical authorities pressured manufacturers to reduce vitamin D doses, claiming toxicity
- Decades of efforts to restrict vitamin D supplementation followed

This hostility persists today, as widespread adoption of high-dose vitamin D3 therapy threatens the profitability of expensive drugs and treatments. The vitamin D3 revolution for MS and other conditions is spreading globally through grassroots efforts, offering hope for affordable and effective treatment options. As more patients experience dramatic improvements, the pressure on mainstream medicine to acknowledge this approach continues to grow.

Back to the VITAL study-a critical examination of the study's design, execution, and interpretation reveals significant flaws that call into question its broad conclusions. Rather than accepting these results at face value, it's essential for healthcare providers, researchers, and the public to approach vitamin D research with a critical eye. As we move forward, it's crucial to: Remain vigilant about potential conflicts of interest in nutrition research and public health recommendations.

Dr. Bruce Hollis's research on vitamin D3 metabolism has shed light on important aspects of how this nutrient functions in the body through two distinct systems: the endocrine system and the autocrine/paracrine system. His work highlights a critical misunderstanding in the scientific community that has led to many flawed study designs and interpretations of vitamin D3 supplementation effects. Now-How has Big Medicine and Big Pharma allegedly tried to suppress the use of adequate doses of vitamin D by the public since the 1920s:

The Suppression of Vitamin D: A Historical Perspective

1920s: The Beginning of Suppression
- In the 1920s, it is claimed that overbuilt for-profit private hospitals began to empty as vitamin D supplementation and sunlight therapy became popular for treating various diseases. Vitamin D was being

added to all sorts of things from beer to hot dogs! It was a craze.

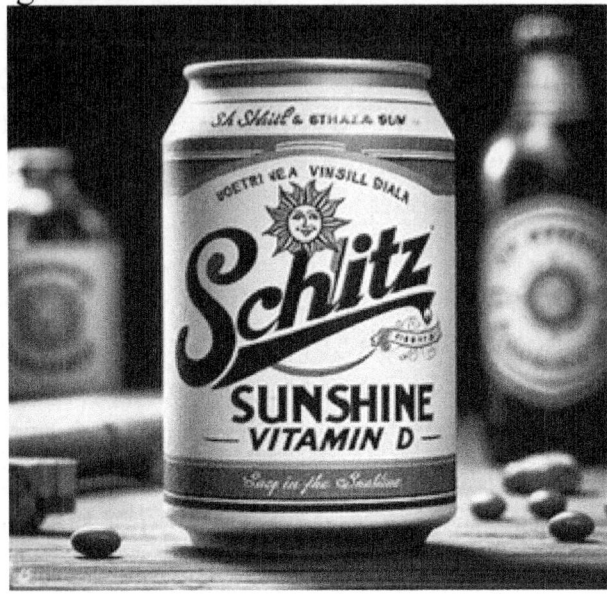

Schlitz beer can from 1928

- This trend allegedly threatened the profitability of the for-profit medical industry, leading to efforts to discredit and suppress vitamin D therapy.

Hospital Capacity and General Population, 1872-1932

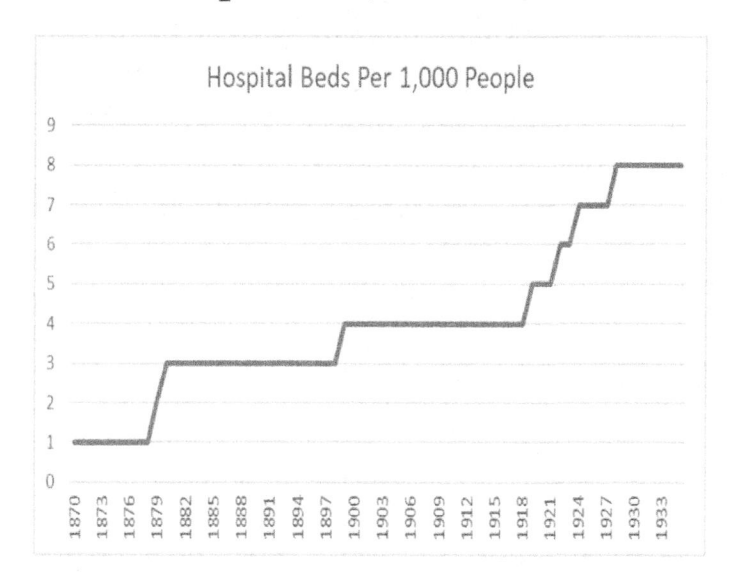

Hospital Beds Per 1,000 People

Data Source: "Hospital Service in the United States: Twelfth Annual Presentation of Hospital Data by the Council on Medical Education and Hospitals of the American Medical Association," *JAMA 100*, 12(March 25, 1933)

Ongoing Conspiracy?

An ongoing conspiracy involving several key aspects:

1. Dosage Misinformation: Deliberate promotion of inadequate vitamin D

dosages to prevent the public from experiencing its full benefits. In the 1920's people were often taking 25 mg of vitamin D3 per day and said to be staying very healthy. This amount was recalibrated by science to become 1 million international units! From 1940 on, the public was then brainwashed into believing any amount over 400 IUs was dangerous and could lead to vitamin D toxicity! 400 IUs was just enough vitamin D needed to be given to a baby to prevent them from getting Rickets (or bow legs). All this was going on while big medicine had created some patented/branded cancer medicines (Drisdol and Deltalin) that were nothing more than pills containing 50,000 IUs of vitamin D.
2. Discourage people's use of sun "health" lamps that actually worked by producing vitamin D in one's skin by rebranding them as quack medical devices.

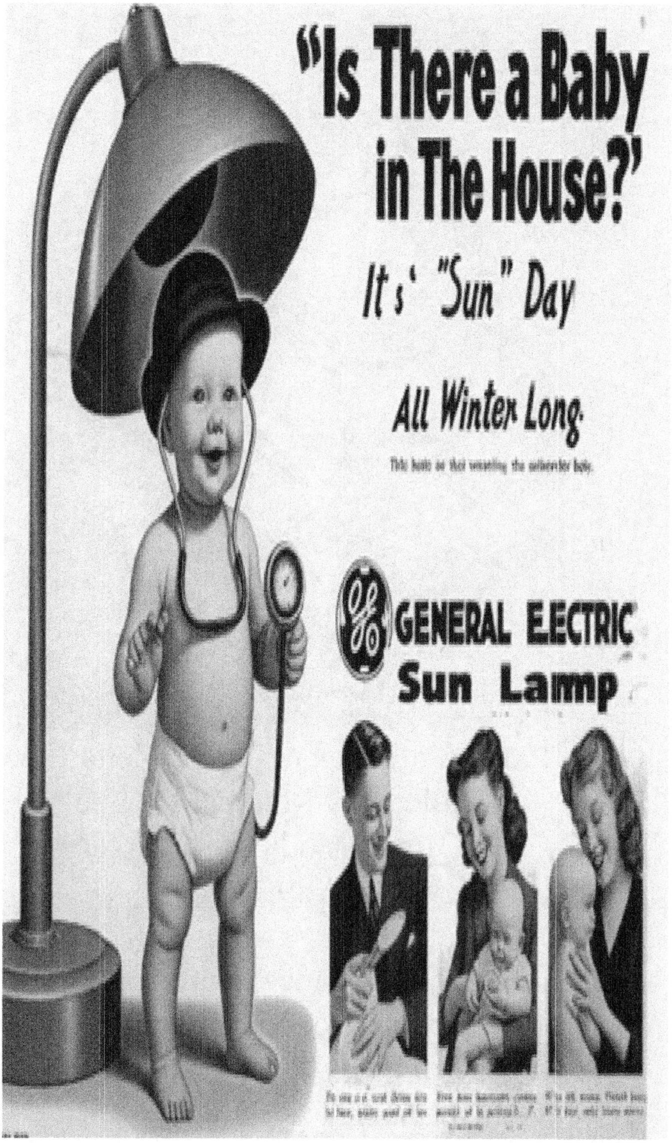
"Is There a Baby
in The House?"
It s' "Sun" Day
All Winter Long.
GENERAL E.ECTRIC
Sun Lamp

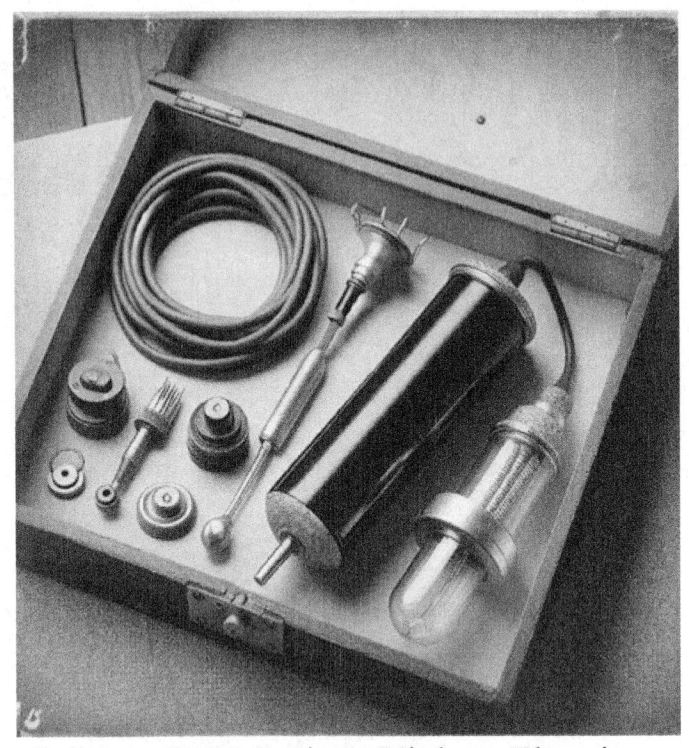

For Sale on eBay: Antique Violetta Electric
Violet Ray Medical Device
<u>Quack</u> Medicine & Box
$29.99

3. Sunlight Avoidance: Campaigns encouraging excessive sun avoidance and sunscreen use, limiting natural vitamin D production.
4. Research Manipulation: Funding of studies designed to show little or no benefit from vitamin D supplementation, often using

insufficient doses. (like the fraudulent VITAL study!)
5. Medical Education: Limiting education on vitamin D's benefits in medical schools, ensuring doctors remain uninformed about its potential.
6. Regulatory Obstacles: Creating regulatory hurdles for high-dose vitamin D supplements and therapies. Big Pharma has been trying to outlaw high dose Vitamin D3 supplements for decades!
7. Media Influence: Using media outlets to spread fear about vitamin D "toxicity" and downplay its benefits.
8. Economic Motivations: Maintaining a population with chronic diseases that require ongoing pharmaceutical treatments is GREAT FOR BUSINESS! Maybe up to 90% of the medical industry would be unnecessary if optimal vitamin D levels were achieved in the population.

Key Players

Various entities implicated in this alleged conspiracy:
- Pharmaceutical companies-the main villains
- Medical associations like Institute of Medicine (IOM) renamed

National Academy of Medicine (NAM) in 2015.
- Medical /Science Journals: JAMA, NEJM, Science, Nature, BMJ etc.
- Government health agencies and Medical Associations: NIH, CDC, Institute of Medicine (IOM) -now known as the National Academy of Medicine, Food and Drug Administration (FDA). World Health Organization (WHO) European Food Safety Authority (EFSA) Health Canada Australian and New Zealand governments
- Researchers at some academic institutions: HARVARD (home of the VITAL study) and many others like Tufts, University of Wisconsin, Yale, UCLA, Oxford, and various universities in New Zealand, Canada, Norway, and Turkey also seem to be in on it.

Consequences

This suppression has led to:
- Widespread vitamin D deficiency
- Increased prevalence of chronic diseases
- Missed opportunities for disease prevention and treatment
- Unnecessary suffering and HUGE healthcare PROFITS!!!

You can see evidence of this continued chronic disease bonanza by just driving around any major metropolitan area. What will you always see: hospitals undergoing large expansion projects, all the time! In fact, in a park by a hospital where I walk my dogs there is always major construction going on and they even put up a bill board …saying "We never stop growing". I was tempted to add, with spray paint, the words, "our bank accounts".

Recognizing and countering this conspiracy could lead to HUGE improvements in public health and a DRAMATIC reduction in the burden of many chronic diseases.

Conclusion: The Vitamin D3 Revolution - Unveiling the Truth and Transforming Health

The shocking ignorance surrounding vitamin D3 has far-reaching consequences on public health, but a paradigm shift is on the horizon. As we unravel the complexities of vitamin D3 metabolism and its dual roles in the endocrine and autocrine/paracrine systems, we stand at the cusp of a health revolution that could transform our approach to disease prevention and treatment.

Correcting Historical Errors

The journey begins with acknowledging and rectifying critical mistakes that have shaped our understanding of vitamin D3:

1. The IOM's Decimal Point Error: The Institute of Medicine's miscalculation led to recommendations that were a mere fraction of what the human body actually needs. This error has perpetuated widespread vitamin D3 deficiency for years.
2. Misunderstanding Vitamin D3 Toxicity: What was once feared as toxicity is now recognized as a deficiency in essential cofactors, primarily magnesium and vitamin K2. This revelation opens the door to higher, more effective dosing strategies.
3. Neglecting the Autocrine System: The focus on the endocrine system has led to flawed study designs and misinterpretations, potentially masking the true benefits of vitamin D3 supplementation.

Unleashing the Power of Optimal Vitamin D3 Levels

The potential impact of correcting these misconceptions is staggering:
- Pandemic Prevention: Adequate vitamin D3 levels could have significantly mitigated the COVID-19 pandemic, enhancing immune function and reducing the severity of infections.
- Cancer Prevention: The "latitude effect" observed in cancer rates suggests a powerful role for vitamin D3 in reducing cancer risk, particularly when combined with its cofactors.
- Autoimmune Disease Management: Even the fatally flawed-ulent VITAL study showed a 22% reduction in autoimmune disease incidence with modest vitamin D3 supplementation.
- Metabolic Health: Emerging evidence points to vitamin D3's potential in managing type 2 diabetes and other metabolic disorders.

A New Paradigm for Vitamin D3 Research and Supplementation

To fully harness the power of vitamin D3, we must adopt a new approach:

1. Higher Dosages: Moving beyond the conservative 2,000 IU daily dose to explore the benefits of 5,000-10,000-50,000 IU or more, guided by individual needs and blood level monitoring.
2. Daily Supplementation: Recognizing the importance of the autocrine system and providing consistent daily doses rather than infrequent large boluses.
3. Cofactor Integration: Ensuring adequate levels of magnesium, vitamin K2, boron, zinc, and vitamin A to optimize vitamin D3 metabolism and effectiveness.
4. Personalized Approaches: Tailoring supplementation strategies based on individual factors such as baseline levels, BMI, age, and genetic variations.
5. Comprehensive Testing: Moving beyond simple 25(OH)D measurements to assess free vitamin D levels and vitamin D binding protein status.

Overcoming Obstacles and Vested Interests

The path forward is not without challenges. The influence of pharmaceutical companies, sunscreen manufacturers, and other vested interests has contributed to the suppression of vitamin D3's true potential. Studies like VITAL have been used to discourage vitamin D3 supplementation **and hinder further research funding**. However, the tide is turning. As more healthcare providers, researchers, and individuals become aware of the limitations of current studies and the vast potential of optimal vitamin D3 levels, a grassroots revolution is taking shape.

A Call to Action

The time has come for a radical reassessment of vitamin D3's role in human health. We must:
1. Demand more rigorous, well-designed studies that account for the complexities of vitamin D3 metabolism and requirement for cofactors.
2. Educate healthcare providers and the public about the true nature of vitamin D3 toxicity and the importance of cofactors.
3. Advocate for updated public health policies that reflect the latest understanding of vitamin D3's role in disease prevention.
4. Empower individuals to take control of their vitamin D3 status through regular testing and personalized supplementation strategies.

The Future of Health

As we correct the shocking ignorance surrounding vitamin D3, we open the door to a future where:
- Autoimmune diseases become rare occurrences rather than lifelong burdens.
- Cancer rates plummet, particularly in regions far from the equator.
- Infectious diseases, including future pandemics, are met with resilient immune systems.
- Metabolic disorders are prevented or reversed through simple, cost-effective interventions.

The vitamin D3 revolution is not just about a single nutrient – it's about recognizing the profound impact that optimal nutrition can have on human health. By embracing this new paradigm, we have the potential to dramatically reduce the burden of chronic disease, enhance quality of life, and reshape the landscape of global health. The journey to unlock the full potential of vitamin D3 has only just begun. As we continue to research, educate, and implement these findings, we stand on the brink of a health transformation that could benefit billions of lives worldwide. The time for action is now – let the vitamin D3 revolution begin.

Appendix A- Fixing our Soils

The Hidden Epidemic: Soil Mineral Deficiencies

America's soils are suffering from a silent crisis that's affecting our health in profound ways. Decades of intensive farming practices have depleted our soils of crucial minerals, leading to widespread deficiencies in magnesium, boron, zinc and others. These deficiencies are not just agricultural problems – they're public health emergencies.

Magnesium: The Forgotten Mineral

Magnesium deficiency in U.S. soils has far-reaching consequences for human health:
- 80%+ of Americans consume less than the required amount of magnesium from food
- Low magnesium levels are associated with type 2 diabetes, metabolic syndrome, hypertension, soft tissue calcification, mitral valve prolapse, cardiovascular disease, heart arrythmias, blood pressure changes, cachexia, many neurological issues including anxiety, panic attacks, concussions, hallucinations, and even death.

- Magnesium deficiency may also contribute to osteoporosis, migraine headaches, and asthma.

Boron: The Arthritis Assassin

Boron deficiency in soils is linked to several health issues:
- Areas with low boron in soil and water supplies have significantly higher rates of arthritis
- Boron supplementation has shown promise in alleviating osteoarthritis symptoms
- Low boron intake affects bone health and vitamin D metabolism
- Regular users of boron are said to have bones so hard that it is difficult for doctors to cut through them

In the 1960s, Dr. Rex Newnham, a plant botanist, made a fascinating discovery that would challenge our understanding of arthritis. While studying soil composition and its effects on plant health, Newnham noticed an intriguing pattern: areas with boron-rich soils had significantly lower rates of arthritis among the population. Newnham's curiosity was piqued when he observed that in regions where daily boron intake was typically 1 mg or less due to soil depletion, the incidence of arthritis ranged from a staggering 20% to 70% of the population. The same rates of arthritis were also seen in the local dogs.

In stark contrast, areas where food was grown in boron rich soils people consumed 3 to 10 mg of boron daily saw arthritis rates plummet to a mere 0% to 10%. And the same was true with their dogs.

This observation led Newnham on a personal journey of discovery. When he moved to Australia, an area with boron-poor soil, to study plants, he developed arthritis himself. Determined to find a solution, he created a simple supplement containing 3 mg of boron. The results were astonishing – not only did he cure his own arthritis, but he found that about 70% of people who tried his boron supplement in Australia reported significant improvement in their arthritis symptoms.

Newnham's findings were so compelling that he presented them at the International Symposium on Trace Elements in Man and Animals in Perth, Australia, in 1981.

He proposed that boron could be an essential micronutrient for humans, particularly in relation to bone and joint health. However, Newnham's discovery was met with resistance from the medical establishment. In a twist of irony, his inexpensive and effective arthritis treatment led to boron being classified as a poison in Australia, effectively banning his supplement. Despite this setback, Newnham's work laid the groundwork for future research into the role of boron in human health, challenging our understanding of nutrition and disease prevention.

Zinc: The Immune System Booster

Zinc deficiency is an emerging global health issue with serious implications:
- Approximately two billion people worldwide are affected by zinc deficiency.
- Low zinc levels can lead to impaired immune function, increased risk of infections, and delayed wound healing.
- Zinc deficiency may contribute to oxidative stress and chronic inflammation.
- Zinc deficiency is thought to be the #1 factor in the cause of sudden infant death syndrome.

A Soil Restoration Plan for RFK Jr.?

To address these critical mineral deficiencies and improve public health, Robert F. Kennedy Jr. could implement the following nationwide plan:
1. National Soil Health Initiative

- Launch a comprehensive program to test and map soil mineral content across the U.S.
- Create targeted strategies for different regions based on specific deficiencies.

2. Regenerative Agriculture Incentives
    - Provide tax breaks and subsidies for farmers who adopt regenerative practices that improve soil health.
    - Encourage crop rotation, cover cropping, and reduced tillage to naturally replenish soil minerals.
3. Mineral Supplementation Program
    - Develop a national program to supplement agricultural soils with magnesium, boron, and zinc based on regional needs.
    - Offer grants to farmers for implementing mineral supplementation strategies.
4. Research and Development Funding
    - Allocate federal funds for research into innovative soil remineralization techniques.
    - Support studies on the long-term effects of soil mineral restoration on public health.
5. Education and Outreach

- Create a public awareness campaign about the importance of soil health and its impact on food quality and human health.
- Develop educational programs for farmers, agronomists, and health professionals on mineral deficiencies and their consequences.

6. Food Labeling Reform
    - Implement new labeling requirements that indicate the mineral content of foods.
    - Create a "Soil Health Certified" label for products grown in mineral-rich soils.

7. School and Community Garden Program
    - Fund the creation of school and community gardens nationwide, emphasizing soil health and mineral-rich produce.
    - Use these gardens as educational tools to teach about nutrition and sustainable agriculture.

8. Biofortification Initiatives
    - Support research and implementation of crop biofortification to increase mineral content in staple foods.

9. Soil Health Monitoring System

- Establish a national database to track soil mineral levels over time.
- Use this data to inform policy decisions and adjust restoration efforts as needed.

10. International Cooperation
   - Collaborate with other countries facing similar soil depletion issues to share knowledge and resources.
   - Lead global efforts to address mineral deficiencies in soils worldwide.

By implementing this comprehensive plan, RFK Jr. could spearhead a revolution in soil health that would have far-reaching benefits for public health, agricultural sustainability, and food security. Restoring our soils to their mineral-rich state is not just an agricultural imperative – it's a crucial step towards creating a healthier, more resilient nation.

Appendix B- Either Outlaw the Feeding of Corn
to Our Livestock or Require Fortification

Either Outlaw the Feeding of Corn to Our Livestock or Require Fortification with a vitamin K1-rich additive, such as alfalfa meal or dried nettle leaves and chlorophyll rich summer grass or grass extracts.

Vitamin K2 deficiency can lead to a wide range of health issues across different age groups and body systems. Here's a detailed look at the health conditions associated with insufficient K2 intake:

Dental and Skeletal Issues
Crooked Teeth in Children

Vitamin K2 plays a crucial role in proper facial and dental development. In children with K2 deficiency:

- The jawbone may not develop to its full potential, leading to overcrowding of teeth

- Inadequate calcium deposition in dental structures can result in weaker teeth more prone to cavities and decay
- The palate may not form properly, potentially causing breathing issues and sleep apnea later in life

Osteoporosis

K2 deficiency can significantly impact bone health:

- Osteocalcin, a K2-dependent protein, is not properly activated, leading to reduced calcium deposition in bones
- This results in decreased bone mineral density and increased fracture risk
- Postmenopausal women are particularly vulnerable to this effect

Cardiovascular Issues-

Arterial Calcification

One of the most significant impacts of K2 deficiency is on cardiovascular health:

- Without sufficient K2, calcium is not properly directed to bones and teeth

- Instead, calcium can accumulate in soft tissues, particularly arteries
- This leads to hardening of arteries (atherosclerosis), increasing the risk of heart disease and stroke

Varicose Veins

K2 deficiency may contribute to the development of varicose veins:

- Calcification of veins can occur, weakening vein walls
- This can lead to the unsightly and uncomfortable bulging associated with varicose veins

Cancer Risk-

Prostate Cancer

K2 deficiency has been linked to an increased risk of prostate cancer:

- A study found that increased K2 intake was associated with a 35% reduction in prostate cancer risk
- The effect was even more pronounced for advanced prostate cancer, with a 63% risk reduction

- In fact, the initiation event for prostate cancer was shown to be calcification of the peripheral zone of the prostate in one study.
- One study showed that men who drank milk (high in calcium) were more likely to get prostate cancer, while those who drank skim milk were at highest risk. Why? Vitamin k2 is found in the fat of the milk when it is present. (This suggests a requirement for dairy farmers to fortify their milk with vitamin K2 would be prudent.)

Other Cancers
While more research is needed, K2 deficiency may increase the risk of other cancers:
- Some studies have shown potential benefits of K2 in reducing the risk of liver cancer recurrence
- K2's role in proper calcium metabolism may help prevent cellular mutations that lead to cancer

Other Health Issues

Kidney Stones
K2 deficiency can contribute to kidney stone formation:
- Without proper K2 levels, matrix-GLA protein remains inactive
- This protein helps prevent calcium accumulation in the kidneys
- K2 deficiency may lead to increased risk of kidney stone formation, especially in those with chronic kidney disease

Diabetes
Emerging research suggests a potential link between K2 deficiency and diabetes:
- K2 may play a role in insulin sensitivity and glucose metabolism
- Some studies indicate that K2 supplementation might help improve insulin sensitivity, though more research is needed

Brain Health
K2 deficiency may impact neurological health:
- K2-dependent proteins play roles in the central and peripheral nervous systems
- Adequate K2 levels may help prevent oxidative stress in the brain

- K2 deficiency could potentially contribute to cognitive decline, though more research is needed in this area

How K2 Deficiency Causes Health Issues

Vitamin K2's primary function is to activate specific proteins that regulate calcium in the body. When K2 is deficient:

- Osteocalcin remains inactive, preventing proper calcium deposition in bones and teeth
- Matrix-GLA protein is not activated, failing to prevent calcium from accumulating in soft tissues
- This leads to a paradoxical situation where bones become weaker while arteries and other soft tissues become calcified
- The body's ability to regulate calcium metabolism is severely impaired, affecting multiple organ systems

By ensuring adequate K2 intake, many of these health issues can potentially be prevented or mitigated. It's important to note that K2 works synergistically with other nutrients, particularly vitamins D3 and A, so a balanced approach to nutrition is key for optimal health.

Feeding corn-based diets to livestock has a significant impact on their vitamin K2 production, which in turn affects the nutritional quality of their milk and tissues. Here's a detailed analysis of this issue and

A proposed plan to address the vitamin K2 issue:

Impact of Corn-Based Diets on Vitamin K2 Production
Corn-based diets virtually eliminate the production of vitamin K2 in livestock for several reasons:

1. Lack of vitamin K1: Corn is low in vitamin K1 (phylloquinone), which animals convert to K2 (menaquinone).
2. Absence of chlorophyll: Corn lacks the high chlorophyll content found in green grass, which is crucial for vitamin K1 synthesis.
3. Limited microbial fermentation: Corn-based diets alter the rumen microbiome, reducing the bacterial populations responsible for converting K1 to K2

The Role of Green Summer Grass

Animals grazing on lush summer pastures produce significantly more vitamin K2 because:
1. High vitamin K1 content: Green grass is rich in vitamin K1, providing the necessary precursor for K2 production.
2. Chlorophyll abundance: Summer grass contains ample chlorophyll, which is essential for vitamin K1 synthesis.
3. Optimal rumen conditions: Grazing on diverse pastures promotes a healthy rumen microbiome, enhancing K1 to K2 conversion.

Winter Grass Deficiencies

Even grass-fed animals may have lower K2 levels in winter due to:
1. Reduced chlorophyll: Winter grass contains less chlorophyll, leading to lower vitamin K1 synthesis.
2. Decreased plant diversity: Winter pastures often have less variety, potentially impacting rumen microbial populations.

3. Lower overall nutrient density: Winter grass generally has lower nutritional value compared to summer grass.

Proposed Plan for Nationwide Implementation

To address the vitamin K2 deficiency in corn-fed livestock, RFK Jr. could propose the following plan:
1. Mandatory Feed Supplementation:
    - Require all corn-based animal feeds to be supplemented with a vitamin K1-rich additive, such as alfalfa meal or dried nettle leaves.
    - Require all corn-based animal feeds to be supplemented with summer grass, chlorophyll, or derivatives.
    - Establish minimum supplementation levels based on animal type and production stage.

2. Pasture Rotation Program:
    - Incentivize farmers to implement rotational grazing systems, allowing animals access to diverse pastures even in confined operations.

- Provide grants for establishing year-round grazing systems with a mix of cool and warm-season grasses.

3. Green Feed Innovation:
    - Fund research into developing indoor "green feed" systems using hydroponic or aeroponic technology to produce chlorophyll-rich feed year-round.
    - Offer tax credits for farmers implementing these systems.

4. Microbial Feed Additives:
    - Develop and promote the use of probiotic feed additives containing K2-producing bacteria to enhance vitamin K2 synthesis in the animal's gut.

5. Education and Training:
    - Launch a nationwide education campaign for farmers on the importance of vitamin K2 in animal nutrition and human health.
    - Provide training on implementing pasture management and feed supplementation strategies.

6. Labeling and Certification:

    - Create a "K2-Rich" certification for animal products meeting specific vitamin K2 content thresholds.
    - Require labeling of vitamin K2 content in dairy and meat products.

7. Research Funding:
    - Allocate federal funds for ongoing research into optimizing vitamin K2 production in livestock and its impact on human health.

8. Monitoring and Enforcement:
    - Establish a national monitoring system to track vitamin K2 levels in animal products.
    - Implement penalties for non-compliance with feed supplementation requirements.

By implementing this comprehensive plan, RFK Jr. could address the vitamin K2 deficiency in corn-fed livestock, improving both animal health and the nutritional quality of animal products for human consumption. This approach aligns with the goal of enhancing the overall health of the nation through improved agricultural practices and nutrition.

Finally, In Case You Were Curious:

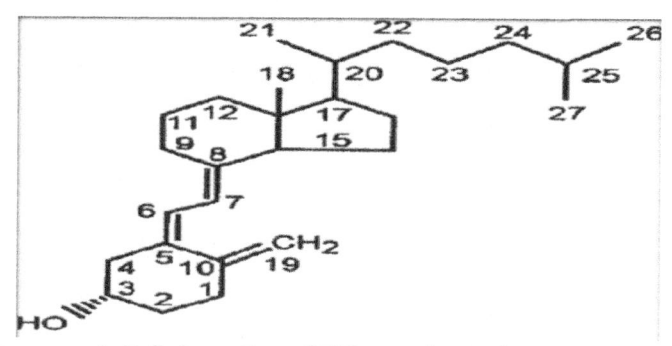

Above- A Molecule of Vitamin D3 With All Its Carbons Numbered

Regular Vitamin D3 (cholecalciferol) has an -OH attached to the 3 carbon.

The more activated form of Vitamin D3 (calcifediol aka calcidiol) has an extra -OH attached to the 25 carbon so it is referred to as 25(OH) D

The most active form of Vitamin D3, calcitriol has a third -OH attached to the 1 Carbon so it is referred to as 1,25 (OH)2 D.

The extra -OHs are needed to allow the D3 to more tightly bind to the Vitamin D receptors, the extra -OHs also make the Vitamin D more polar and soluble which enhances transport in the blood stream and also allows the Vitamin D to interact more with target proteins.

(so technically to be consistent, we should have referred to the three forms as 3 (OH)1 D, 3,25 (OH)2 D and 1, 3, 25 (OH)3 D).. but they love to make things complicated!)